A SOLDIER'S WILL TO LIVE

DEFYING THE ODDS

Abraham Anderson

Edited by Divine Editing & Proofreading Services

Published by Victorious You Press™
Charlotte NC, USA

Copyright © 2024 Abraham Anderson All rights reserved.

No part of this book may be reproduced, distributed or transmitted in any form by any means, graphic, electronic, or mechanical, including photocopy, recording, taping, or by any information storage or retrieval system, without permission in writing from the author except in the case of reprints in the context of reviews, quotes, or references.

While the author has made every effort to ensure that the ideas, statistics, and information presented in this Book are accurate to the best of his/her abilities, any implications direct, derived, or perceived, should only be used at the reader's discretion. The author cannot be held responsible for any personal or commercial damage arising from communication, application, or misinterpretation of the information presented herein.

Unless otherwise indicated, scripture quotations are from the Holy Bible, King James Version. All rights reserved.

TITLE: A SOLDIER'S WILL TO LIVE
First Printed: 2024

Cover Designer: Perfect Design Studios
Editor: Lynn Braxton: Divine Editing & Proofreading Services

ISBN: 978-1-959719-39-7
ISBN: (eBook) 978-1-959719-40-3
Library of Congress Control Number: 2024918610
Printed in the United States of America

For details email joan@victoriousyoupress.com
or visit us at www.victoriousyoupress.com

DEDICATION

To all men and women who have endured tragedies, hardship, pain, loss, and setbacks, choose to follow Christ for your healing.

To married couples who choose to strengthen their relationships, don't give up. Strive for a marriage that is built on Biblical principles and learn to love and respect one another.

To my wife, Annette H. Anderson, and my children, you are my rock!

To my readers, I hope you find God's handy work in these pages encouraging. May you continue to find hope in your future based on God's Word.

ACKNOWLEDGMENT

To my gorgeous wife, Annette H. Anderson, my strong tower and spiritual partner, your unwavering commitment to our marriage and family, especially during my health battles, has been nothing short of heroic. Your love, patience, and faith have been my guiding light, and I am blessed to have you by my side. Thank you for being my rock and my constant source of support.

To my beloved children, Abraham Jamal Anderson, Brandon Rahsaan Anderson, and Tiyauna Chanel Anderson Zambrano, I love and treasure you more than you will ever know. Thank you for the love and support you have given me over the years.

To Joan Randall of Victorious You Press, I extend my deepest gratitude to you and your amazing team for believing in my vision, sharing your ideas on how to execute them, and providing the platform to share my story with the world. Thank you for your support!

To Lynn Braxton, my editor, thank you for your thoughtful advice, creativity, patience, and skillful editing, which contributed to the success of this book. Thank you for your support throughout this writing journey.

To Pastor Art and Kuna Sepulveda, Word of Life Hawaii, thank you for being there to support me and my family and for assigning other pastors to support us while I was going through my illness and healing process. Your leadership taught us the true meaning of being steadfast in God's Word.

To my family, my brother, who traveled to Hawaii, and my sisters, who supported me with their calls, prayers, and cards, I love and appreciate you all. Thank you for also requesting that other church groups, including Trinity Broadcasting Network (TBN), pray for me. I will never forget the support and love they showed me.

To my mother-in-law, Dorothy W. Spriggs, may you rest in Heaven. Thank you for dropping everything to come and assist my wife and care for our children while I was in the hospital.

To the Readers, I thank God for the opportunity to share my testimony with you. I pray that He gives you the ears to hear and the heart to receive what He has in store for you if you just believe in Him.

TABLE OF CONTENTS

Preface	1
Introduction	5
From Mandatory Worship to Personal Faith	11
The Love of My Life	15
Troubled Teen Years	21
A New Beginning	29
Our Journey to Forever!	35
Duty Calls	41
Breaking the Cycle	45
Seeking Comfort in a Bottle	53
A Life-Changing Moment	57
Military Life: From One Duty Station to Another	61
From Aloha to Agony	65
Clinging to Hope: Awaiting the Results	71
Preparing for Warfare	75

PREFACE

I Want to Live: The Battle for My Life

The doctor walked in and greeted us. I took a deep breath, preparing myself for our discussion. His serious expression said everything! This was not going to be good news! Dread quickly enveloped me. I couldn't breathe, and my heart beat so hard I thought it would jump out of my chest. I couldn't take my eyes off the neurologist as he stood in front of us to tell us the results.

His eyes darted from my eyes to my wife's as he reviewed the results of my scans as if it were the morning news, with no emotion in his voice. "The MRI shows you have a massive brain tumor located in the lower back part of your brain called the posterior fossa. This type of tumor is called Ependymoma and can block the flow of spinal fluid and put increased pressure on your brainstem. If that happens, you may experience difficulty walking, including balance issues, nausea, vertigo, and other symptoms. I recommend that we schedule you for an emergency surgery right away."

The news hit hard! I was numb and shocked—rendered speechless! I just stared at the doctor in disbelief. Not only do I have to process the fact that I have a tumor on my brain, but we have to make the decision for me to undergo surgery immediately! My head was whirring, and thoughts were running rapidly through my mind. I didn't know what to say.

"What are the risks with this surgery?" My wife's voice trembled slightly, breaking the silence.

"The good news is that with this type of tumor, there is a 92 percent survival rate depending on the patient's overall health," the doctor began. "However, there are potential risks associated with the surgery that you'll need to consider. Abraham, you present as a very healthy young man who has taken very good care of himself physically," he said, glancing in my direction. Then, he turned and spoke directly to Annette, "But this operation may cause him to have a stroke or experience speech or memory problems. He may lose strength in his legs or suffer paralysis. Abraham may have swelling on the brain or develop a blood clot. He could also lose his life during surgery."

Everything the doctor said blurred together in my mind. His words hung in the air, heavy, suffocating me, fully taking my breath away. I was shocked as I stared at

The Battle Begins	79
Radiation Treatment	87
The Faith To Fight	91
Through Sickness and Health	95
The Strength of the Church	101
A Second Chance	105
An Enduring Love and Eternal Commitment	111
Summary	115
Resources	121
About The Author	123

him, bewildered by the words that spilled out of his mouth, "Stroke, speech problems, paralysis, and possible death." *Is he talking about me? Oh, my God,* I thought. *This can't be real. I've always taken good care of my body. He must be wrong. He said he "suspects" it's a brain tumor, but he doesn't know for sure.* My mind raced, grasping at any possible denial. *It just can't be true. I can't accept that! Not me. I'm healthy. It must be a mistake!*

I sat there, numb, trying to deal with the enormity of the whole situation crashing in on me.

INTRODUCTION

I am Abraham Anderson, the seventh of nine siblings, born and raised in the busy city of Baltimore, Maryland. My childhood was a mix of hardships and invaluable life lessons, shaped by an environment often marred by alcohol and drugs.

My early school experience was a significant challenge for me. As a slow learner, I had difficulty comprehending Basic Math and English assignments. I felt intimidated by my teacher and peers, which made me terrified to participate in classroom activities, particularly those involving peer interactions. My low self-esteem and shyness further exacerbated these issues, affecting my behavior and feelings towards others.

One of the most embarrassing moments in middle school was during a talent show performance with the school rock band. I was very anxious as time neared for my solo part of playing the drums. I started off okay but was horrified when I dropped my drumstick. The entire auditorium went silent. I heard a few gasps as the audience stared at me in shock. My anxiety level skyrocketed, reaching an all-time high. I managed to quickly pull myself together, retrieved the stick, and completed my performance. It was rewarding to hear the thunderous applause for our rock band!

In my spare time after school, I spent many hours with my neighbor, Julius Foster, learning to play chess and spades. These moments made me feel like I was in *my* element and helped me develop my strategic thinking skills.

My parents never read stories to us at bedtime, leaving me unaware of the potential benefits of that experience. Perhaps, if they had, it could have fostered a love for reading and learning from a young age. This ritual might have enhanced my language skills, increased my imagination, and created a comforting and supportive environment. The bonding time could have also built my confidence and curiosity, making me more eager to engage in academic activities and overcome educational challenges.

The importance of education was never emphasized in our home, perhaps because neither of my parents finished middle school. Consequently, pursuing a higher education was never a priority in our household. They never talked to us about the importance of going to college. However, my sister, Tinnie, came to my rescue when she noticed I was struggling with my school's academic requirements. She spent countless hours helping and preparing me for success in higher education. I wouldn't be where I am today without her unwavering commitment and support.

My parents were deeply religious and devoted ministers with distinct beliefs. Their strict religious practices significantly shaped my perspective on life and religion. My sisters were not allowed to wear pants, sleeveless shirts, or makeup. If they did, my parents ridiculed them. We knew there would be hell to pay if we brought a bad report card home. This type of rigidity made me reluctant to embrace church until I found a personal connection with God later in my life.

My father, Benjamin Anderson, had a learning deficit; he never finished elementary school. Yet, he thrived as an auditory learner. He would pay my siblings and me—Tinnie, Benjamin Jr., Joel, and Patricia—to read the Bible to him a day or two before his sermons. He memorized the scriptures and recited them verbatim, making it appear as if he was reading. At church, he would ask a deacon or other member of the congregation to read the scripture. Many in the congregation didn't know he couldn't read. Despite his challenges, he was a devout Christian, traveling across the country to fellowship with other churches and ministries.

He was a provider, doing what it took to ensure our water, lights, heat, and telephone bills were paid. During his early years in the South, he picked cotton and tobacco and even dug graves. He taught us practical skills, too. Every year or two, he would buy a new car, usually an Oldsmobile, which he loved.

My mother, Martha Lee Anderson, was a domestic engineer and a jack of all trades but is not an expert at anything. She gave birth to nine children over a twenty-year span. She was our family's authoritarian, taking control of household responsibilities, including disciplining us since our father did not seem to have the wherewithal to do so. My mother was very strict and sometimes abusive. There were times I had to wear long sleeves to school to hide the whelps and scars from my peers and teachers. My siblings and I were well aware of my mother's sisters making snide remarks and looking down on her for having so many children and focusing on raising them instead of pursuing an education or a reputable job. This may be one of the reasons she took her frustration out on us.

One day, I was playing with the stove when my mother came out of nowhere and caught me. She grabbed my hand and held it on the hot stove until I began to feel the intense heat. No matter how much I screamed and tried to wriggle away from her grasp, yelling, "I'm sorry! I'm sorry! I won't do it again," she was relentless and determined to teach me a lesson. After that, I didn't need any reminders not to play with the stove. Such harsh discipline was a regular part of our upbringing.

FROM MANDATORY WORSHIP TO PERSONAL FAITH

When I was growing up, it was mandatory and non negotiable to attend and be active in the church. My parents, devoted Pentecostal church members, required all nine of their children to attend services at least three times a week. This routine included Sunday school, morning service, night service, and Wednesday night service. Thursday was choir practice—my brother Joseph played the guitar, my mother was a pianist, I played the drums, and my other siblings sang. We went to revivals that could last one or two weeks and traveled to churches throughout Baltimore to fellowship and worship.

Occasionally, we would sneak off to play with our friends and enjoy our time away from the church. But when we got caught, our parents' punishments were swift and harsh, sometimes involving beatings for our defiance.

I vowed that once I moved out, I would not attend church regularly. The numerous restrictions—no movies, no dances or parties, no drinking beer, and only having Christian friends—were considered necessary to avoid sinful behavior and please God. When I finally gained my independence, I felt liberated and acted out against these biblical principles, enjoying the freedom from what I had perceived as oppressive rules.

Despite my initial rebellion, I never lost sight of the values instilled in me. I still honor God's words about my future and strive for success. Now, I attend church regularly, free from the restrictions of my past. This personal journey has allowed me to reconnect with my faith in a more meaningful and self-determined way.

The Holy Church of Power Interstates ordained my mother, qualifying her as a pastor and permitting her to establish her own church. She searched near and far throughout Baltimore for a suitable facility to hold services. However, after looking at numerous buildings that she deemed "holes in the walls," she could not find a building that was sufficient for what she had envisioned. So, my mother decided to convert our living room into a church, much to my father's dismay.

When my father realized what my mother was doing, he was not having it! He began throwing chairs and worship items out the window of our home. News spread quickly about what was going on in the Anderson household. We soon became the laughingstock of the neighborhood.

Nothing deterred my mother from creating her church within our home. She had a plan and wanted to make sure it came to fruition. So, she started raising money for a building fund. My siblings and I had to sell flavored ice cones, candy apples, and bags of popcorn in our driveway.

There was constant turmoil in our home. My siblings and I often found ourselves caught in the middle of our parents' conflicts, which caused significant division among us. Some of my siblings sided with my mother, while others aligned with my father, the family's breadwinner. Overall, their influence, though strict, devout, and religious, left a lasting impression on my views of life and faith.

THE LOVE OF MY LIFE

During an evening service at my mother's church, I was playing the drums. While scanning the audience from my advantage point perched on the pulpit, my eyes fell upon the most beautiful girl I had ever seen. She was sitting in the back row—chatting with someone who looked like she could be her sister. I could not stop gazing at her. She was stunning. Her beauty took my breath away, sending a warm shiver down my spine. The palms of my hands began to sweat. I struggled to stay focused on the song I was playing on my drums. I could hardly wait for the service to end. As time ticked by slowly, I hoped to muster up the courage to greet her.

As the service concluded and everyone started mingling, I took a deep breath and walked toward her, my heart pounding so loud I thought someone might hear it.

"Hi, I'm Abraham," I said, trying to steady my voice. "I noticed you during the service. What is your name?"

She looked up at me with a warm smile. "Hi, Abraham, I'm Annette. It's nice to meet you. This is my sister, Lydia."

"Hi." I nodded in Lydia's direction, then quickly shifted my gaze back to Annette. Despite my shy nature, I pressed on. "Would it be alright if we talked for a bit?"

"Sure," she replied, her eyes sparkling. "I'd like that."

During our conversation, I felt a bit uneasy, wondering whether my mix of nervousness and excitement was coming off as too aggressive. However, Annette didn't seem to be put off and kept smiling as we talked. Annette was thirteen, and I was fifteen. She seemed very comfortable talking with me. The connection between us was undeniable.

My High School Love

During our high school years at Mergenthal Vocational Technical High School, we were able to talk on the telephone more. We spent countless hours talking about our daily lives and dreaming of the next time we'd see each other. In those days of rotary phones and shared party lines, we would talk until my mother or siblings told us to get off the phone. I was captivated by her. Our conversations were filled with hopes and future plans.

I told Annette I would love to visit her. She checked with her parents to make sure it was okay to tell me where she lived. They gave her permission, and she rattled off the address. I was so excited that my stomach felt as if it were filled with butterflies. I immediately jumped on my bicycle and rode all the way to her house. She lived about fifteen miles, which took about thirty minutes from my door to hers.

When I finally met her parents for the first time, they extended me a warm welcome. Both our families were Christians, making it easier to bond with them. They embraced me with open arms. I felt comfortable talking to them.

One evening, as we sat talking, I knew it was the perfect time to ask Annette the question that had been on my mind for so long. Taking a deep breath, I held her hand and looked into her eyes. "Annette, would you be my girlfriend?"

The biggest smile spread across her face, "Yes," she said as her eyes sparkled.

From that moment on, we were so fascinated with one another that we were inseparable, trying to spend as much time together as possible. Annette became interested in nursing and began attending the same high school I was enrolled in. I'll never forget the first time I saw her walking down the hall. I was mesmerized! She looked as gorgeous as the first day I met her. And because I cherished every opportunity I could spend with Annette, I often skipped one of my classes to see her during her lunch period.

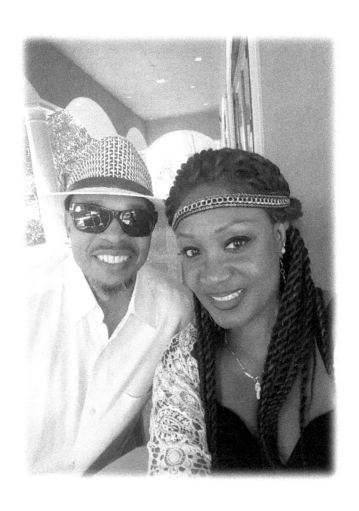

TROUBLED TEEN YEARS

When I was in high school, I tended to mimic the inappropriate behaviors I witnessed around me. One pivotal day during the summer, I decided to purchase marijuana from a neighbor. After giving him ten dollars, he handed me the smallest dime bag I had ever seen. I was upset and called him out on it. I didn't know why he was trying to cheat me. Things quickly got out of hand and escalated into a violent altercation right in front of my house.

My neighbor pulled out a knife, and I grabbed my baseball bat. We faced off against each other—neither of us wanted to back down, so we began to swing our weapons at one another. In the midst of the struggle, I felt his knife puncture the layers of skin, sinking deep into the folds of my right abdomen. I grimaced and gasped for breath. I couldn't believe he stabbed me. Before I could do anything to defend myself, he quickly yanked the knife out and stabbed me again–this time in my upper right arm. The pain was excruciating as it radiated up and down my arm.

"I have to fight back! I have to defend myself, or he's going to kill me," the thoughts raced through my mind. I swung the bat, hitting him in the head. Exhausted from the battle and our wounds, we both stopped fighting. I looked down; blood was everywhere. My neighbor didn't get away injury-free; he was hurt, too. Someone called an ambulance; they took me to the hospital, where I had to stay for three days.

The doctor said the stab wound to my torso was very close to my ribs but didn't cause any damage to the rib cage. However, the injury to my upper arm resulted in severe nerve damage, causing significant health challenges, including the ability to open and close my hand, and left me with limited mobility in that arm, ultimately ending my football aspirations.

However, I didn't allow my limitations to deter me from pursuing athletics. I joined my high school's cross-country team, which boosted my morale and provided a sense of accomplishment. Only the names of the top five to finish the run would have their names announced on the intercom. I smiled and was especially proud of myself when I heard my name called over the school intercom the next day.

At home, my living conditions were dire. Roach and rat infestations, plus the stench of their decaying bodies within the walls permeating our home, were almost too much to bear. Our family relied on federal assistance, which meant eating government cheese, consuming powdered milk, sometimes containing small bugs, and receiving some fruit and vegetables that were rotten and not edible. This was no way to live, but it was our reality.

In the fall, many kids looked forward to the start of a new school year because they could go shopping for new clothes. However, my siblings and I didn't have that luxury. We had to wear each other's hand-me-down clothes, some with holes in them, yet another sign that we were poor. We didn't think much about it, though, because it was just the way things were when we were growing up. Ironically, today, it is deemed fashionable to wear clothes designed with holes.

During the winter season, when the temperature dropped below freezing, it was particularly harsh on our family. We often ran out of oil to heat our home and couldn't afford to buy more. In order to stay as warm as we could, our father showed us how to boil water on the stove, which created steam. As a result, the steam helped to warm the house.

Despite these hardships, my educational journey offered glimpses of a better future. During the desegregation era, I was bused to an all-white school, where the curriculum, books, and technology were superior to what I had known. However, my siblings attended a different school and often ridiculed me, telling me I had "the brawn but not the brains." This cruelty only fueled my determination to excel academically and professionally.

Broken Rules

One night, during my high school years, I returned home from hanging out with friends to find the front door locked. I tried to unlock it, to no avail. It was bolted—there was no way I was getting inside tonight. "Dang! I missed my curfew!" I said, exhaling a long, slow breath. Tired and exasperated, I tried banging on the front door, but my knocks went unanswered. Cold and hungry with nowhere to go, I had to sleep on the porch in the freezing rain and snow with only my coat to keep me warm.

As I lay on the porch, exposed to the elements and shivering uncontrollably, I questioned why this was happening to me. Angry and frustrated, I thought, *This is abuse! Why would someone subject their child to this? What did I do to make them so angry that they don't even care if I freeze to death? Do my parents love me? If they did, why do I feel unwanted, so dejected, and unloved?* I know I'm not a bad kid; I just need guidance.

In the morning, I heard the lock click. One of my siblings opened the door, looking at me with pity. I jumped up, dashed inside, thankful to be out of the cold elements. I was still shaking and looking forward to wrapping myself in something warm, but before I could go to my room, my mother blocked me with her body.

With arms crossed, she said sternly, "Abraham, all you had to do was follow my rules, and you would have been in this warm house with everybody else. Staying out late with your buddies is not acceptable. So, don't let it happen again."

You would think I had learned my lesson after having to sleep on the porch in the freezing cold. I admit I continued to test the boundaries, knowing my mother was a strict disciplinarian. During my senior year in high school, my mother apparently had enough of my antics and failure to follow her rules. One day, she looked at me and said, "Since you can't seem to follow my rules, you have to get out."

"What? You're kicking me out? Mom, please! Where am I supposed to go?" I asked, pleading for mercy.

"Since you want to act like you're grown, you figure it out."

I stood there shocked, staring at my mother in disbelief. I knew she did not believe in sparing the rod, but I never thought she would kick me out of the only home I have ever known. My heart sank as the reality of her words hit me. *I guess I tested the boundaries too many times*, I thought.

I was often upset with my mother, but I had to acknowledge that my behavior and lifestyle were not up to her standards. Still, I wasn't sure what I was going to do when she told me I had to get out of our home for staying out late with my friends. I thought she would put me on punishment or whip me. I didn't think she would ever put me out of our house. I'm too young to get a place of my own. Where am I supposed to go? Who will take me in?

As I contemplated my next steps, the only solution I could come up with was to ask my older sister, Patricia, if I could stay with her. I called and explained what had happened. She talked to her then-husband, David Evans, and they agreed I could live there until I finished high school. They told me in order to stay under their roof, I had to get my act together.

I put myself in this unexpected predicament and had to move about forty-five minutes away. Even though this was not what I expected to happen in my life, I found joy in the midst of my crisis because my childhood sweetheart, Annette, lived only a block from my sister.

A NEW BEGINNING

In 1978, I was excited when I completed my high school requirements and was able to graduate. What a relief when I stood with my diploma in my hand. I could finally exhale. *I did it!* I thought with so much pride in my heart. I knew this was a pivotal moment for me. Annette still had one more year before she was eligible to graduate.

Amidst my celebration of being out of high school, a significant decision weighed on my mind—what am I going to do with my future? Now that I was considered an adult, I needed to figure out what to do with my life. I knew I didn't want to end up like some of my friends who were either incarcerated, strung out on drugs, or dead. I wasn't sure if I had the skills to make a living on my own. So, I decided to ask my brother-in-law, David, for guidance on this matter. He seemed eager to talk to me about future opportunities if I enlisted in the military. We discussed the pros and cons. Following a long discussion, he persuaded me to join the United States Army.

Duty Calls: Taking the Oath

Within a couple of weeks, I went to talk to a recruiter who explained that I had to complete an entrance test and pass a physical exam. I had to pass the Armed Services Vocational Aptitude Battery, a written test called the ASVAB, which determined which job I qualified for.

After passing the required tests, I had to take an oath and swear to support and defend the Constitution of the United States, bear allegiance to it, and obey orders given by my superiors. While signing the papers, I was ecstatic and nervous at the same time but so honored to perform my duty. This was a huge, life-changing decision, but I knew it was the best decision I could make for my life.

I wasn't sure how Annette would feel about me going into the military. She was the love of my life, and I didn't want to do anything that would cause her anguish. So, the next day, I went to talk to her about the decision I made.

"Annette, I know it will be tough on you with me leaving for basic training," I said, "but I promise you that every day I'm away from you, I will be working towards building our future. I have to do this for myself and for us. That's the only reason I enlisted."

Initially, I could tell she was sad and a bit upset because I had sprung this news on her. She acknowledged that it concerned her because we would be separated while I went to basic training. However, she stated she was proud of me and supported my decision because she knew it was the right one for me at the time.

Annette nodded, her resolve strengthening. "I understand, and I'll be here waiting for you. We'll write letters and call whenever we can, and before you know it, we'll be together again. I believe in you, Abraham, and I believe in us."

Before leaving for Basic Training, I had another important task to do. Despite our differences, I knew it was important for me to tell my mother about my plans. So, I went by her house to share my news. I told her I would be leaving for Basic Training, and she agreed to meet me at the train station to say goodbye.

Embracing the Call to Duty

The day I left for Basic Training was one of the hardest days for Annette and me. We hugged tightly. "I love you," I whispered, my voice cracking as I thought about the time I would need to be away from my love. "I'll be back before you know it," I said, trying to reassure her.

Annette clung to me as if her heart were aching with our impending separation. "I love you too, Abraham. Stay safe, and remember, we're in this together."

A few days later, when I arrived at the train station, I spotted my mother and headed in her direction. We talked briefly and hugged, and then she wished me well. I stepped on the train as she turned and walked away. I loved my mother but never had a close relationship with her because of her stringent, tough-love mentality.

Weeks turned into months as I endured the rigors of training. Letters became our lifeline, filled with words of love, encouragement, and dreams of our life together. Annette counted down the days until my return, each letter and phone call fueling our hope and determination.

Transitioning to Military Life

Enlisting in the Army provided me an escape from the troubled environment of my youth. I quickly embraced the discipline and structure of military life. I spent eight weeks at Fort Dix, New Jersey, the basic training post, whose main goal was to turn thousands of civilians like me into top-rate soldiers. The training also prepared me to understand the Army structure and procedures I had to follow during military assignments.

Next, I was sent to Advanced Individual Training (AIT) for three months at Fort Polk, Louisiana, to equip me with the skills needed for my new career. I trained as a

Physical Activity Specialist, which covered a variety of career strategies and standards for the job opportunities available. Later, I transitioned to the role of a Veterinary Food Inspector, where I ensured the safety and quality of food supplies, a role critical to maintaining the health of fellow soldiers.

My military career took me to various duty stations, including Fort Eustis, Virginia, where I was a physical fitness trainer. Then, I went to Fort Greely, Alaska, where I worked at the Youth Activity Center. Each assignment brought new responsibilities, from rehabilitating soldiers to developing youth programs.

OUR JOURNEY TO FOREVER!

Annette and I had been in a courtship for over six years and had many conversations about wanting to get married and live together. I was elated that I had the privilege of building a relationship with her parents. During this time, both of our families had the opportunity to meet, and they all approved our decision to marry.

Finally, the day arrived when I completed Basic Training and was able to go home. Only one thing was on my heart and mind: to reconnect with Annette. I had already decided that she was truly the one I wanted to spend the rest of my life with. So, I went to her house, ready to ask for her hand in marriage. Even though we had talked about getting married, she had no idea I would be asking her to marry me that day.

We were so excited to finally see each other. We chatted for a few minutes, then the mood became serious as I looked at her intently, "Annette," I said, as I tried to steady my voice despite the adrenaline surging through me, "we've shared so many dreams together, and I want to start making them a reality." I took a deep breath, dropped to one knee, pulled the box out of my pocket, and presented the ring to her. I could see the excitement in her eyes. My heart was beating fast as I took in a deep breath and asked, "Would you be my wife?"

Her eyes beamed with excitement, and her hands trembled as she covered her mouth. "Oh, Abraham," she whispered, overwhelmed with emotion. She seemed so excited as she joyfully said, "Yes!"

We embraced, sealing our commitment with a kiss that spoke volumes of our shared history and future. We were both happy beyond measure. I was truly ecstatic because it seemed that she truly believed in me. We were both on cloud nine, as they say. We smiled and laughed the rest of the day.

After being on leave for a week, I had to return to my duty station. I knew how important it was for us to stay connected during my time away from Annette, so we had agreed to frequent phone calls and writing letters. Early on, we wrote to one another once a month and talked on the phone regularly, continuing to express our love and commitment. But I soon fell into a lapse in my judgment and quit writing Annette for about three months. I wasn't sure why I let this happen. I knew how much I loved her, and she loved me. But after so much time had passed, I was scared that our relationship wouldn't survive.

Finally, I got up the nerve and called her to apologize. My heart pounded as I waited for her to answer the phone. After a few rings, she picked up the phone.

"Hello," she said, flatly without emotion.

I could tell right away that she was irritated with me. I chose my words carefully, but I knew I had wronged her and didn't want to cause any more problems or distrust.

"Annette, I'm so sorry. I know I have been irresponsible in not calling you and keeping in touch.

Initially, she was very upset and didn't hesitate to tell me what she thought about my actions. At one point, she said she was so angry that I was not contacting her that she threw the engagement ring across the room. After a long discussion, I was so relieved when she said she forgave me.

After leaving Alaska, I was assigned to Fort Ritchie in Maryland. Annette and I started planning so we could be married. We discussed where we wanted to have our ceremony. I suggested the courthouse; however, Annette was not in agreement with that. She wanted a formal ceremony. So, we agreed to a large church wedding and reception at St. John Alpha & Omega Church in Baltimore, MD. Her Godfather, Pastor Lloyd Hall, agreed to marry us.

In 1982, the day we longed for finally arrived. We stood in the church, ready to be wed in front of our family and friends. My eyes gaped in awe as I saw my beautiful bride coming down the aisle. When she stopped and stood before me, I was humbled to know that she chose me, and I chose her to live out the rest of our days with one another.

Pastor Hall led us through the exchange of our vows. Then, he announced, "You may kiss the bride." I knew this kiss and this moment would be different. Annette was no longer my girlfriend or fiancé; she was my wife. When we kissed, I felt electrified, so excited that our dream finally came true.

It was a day I will never forget as we celebrated our love for one another and our marriage with friends and family. We couldn't stop smiling as we danced and enjoyed good food. We were excited to receive lots of nice gifts to help us set up our new home. We were anxious to start our new life together as husband and wife.

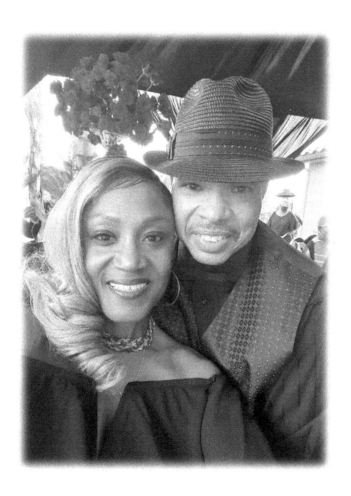

DUTY CALLS

It was finally time to report to my duty station in Annapolis, MD, which was under the command of Fort Meade. Thankfully, my wife was able to join me. The first few months of marriage were interesting as we tried our best to adjust to our new roles as husband and wife. Annette had enrolled in school and was a full-time nursing student and was working full-time, too. I supported her vision of becoming a nurse and did everything I could to show her how proud I was. Although it was hard to balance our work and family life, we put all our effort into making it work. Our family life was so rewarding.

Three years later, I couldn't believe it when Annette announced she was pregnant! I was thrilled, yet scared because I was unsure of my ability to be a good dad. This weighed heavy on my heart. I didn't feel prepared because I had not received any guidance on being a husband or father, and my parents had not been good role models in how to parent children correctly. But my sweet Annette kept reassuring me that I would do fine.

Words cannot express how excited I was the day my first child, a son, Abraham Jamal Anderson, was born. I was in awe of him as I lifted him into my arms for the first time. Annette watched from her hospital bed, smiling. I looked at this bundle of joy, smiling at him— nervously, realizing, "I'm a father." I desperately wanted to be the best dad to him, but I didn't know what I was up against. That's what frightened me. So, I prayed and sought guidance from God. He helped prepare me for one of the most important roles of my life.

From Homeland to Overseas

When I received my Permanent Change of Station (PCS) order to report to my next duty station, West Ruislip Naval Station, in England, my son was around two years old. Unfortunately, I would have to leave my family behind because my duties required that I go through some additional training. This was very difficult for us as a young couple. Annette would have to manage the household on her own. I reassured Annette that she would be able to join me overseas in about six months.

My new job as a procurement Quality Assurance inspector was very interesting. I was responsible for inspecting all the carcasses—beef, lamb, and pork—that were shipped to our base to feed our soldiers, ensuring they met United States standards. These duties were different from anything I had been assigned to do before.

I was so excited and happy when it was finally time for Annette and our son to join me. Before they arrived, I had applied for housing and was approved for British housing for active-duty American soldiers and their families.

Over the next few years, we had two more children born in England—Brandon Rahsaan Anderson and Tiyauna Chanel Anderson. It was a blessing to see our little family grow. Annette is a very spiritual woman, and she and the kids found a church they enjoyed worshipping at. Being around other Christians seemed to bring her peace and joy. I would sometimes, just sit back and smile, taking it all in, seeing my wife and kids so content.

BREAKING THE CYCLE

As my boys grew older, those happy moments changed whenever I had to spank them when they disobeyed our rules. One day, after they were caught playing with matches, I disciplined them. I wanted to teach them a lesson so they wouldn't hurt themselves or burn our house down.

I could tell Annette was not happy with the way I disciplined our children. She hugged them and sent them to their room.

Annette turned toward me, her voice sounding frustrated, "Abe, you can't keep spanking our children. Whipping our children with a belt isn't teaching them anything but fear. We ***will not*** raise our children like you were raised," she said firmly. "Your parents left scars on your body when they beat you. Is that what you want for our children? Do you want our sons to love and respect you, even when you have to discipline them? If you do, you cannot treat them like this. You have to discipline them with love."

The room felt heavy with tension, and the smell of burnt paper filled the air. I looked down, the belt still clutched in my hand. I slowly put it back on, feeding it through the loops of my pants while contemplating everything Annette said.

After our discussion, we went to our sons' room. I stood in the doorway while Annette talked to them. She stooped down until her eyes met theirs. "Boys, do you understand what you did was wrong?"

"Yes!" They said sadly.

"Do you understand why Daddy was upset?" she asked gently.

They nodded and looked in my direction, "Sorry, Daddy!"

I nodded, still unsure if this was really how to discipline our sons.

Annette continued, "Daddy loves you, and he just didn't want either of you to get burned or set our house on fire. Do you understand?"

"Yes."

"Alright!" Annette said, standing while embracing them warmly.

They hugged her as hard as they could while glancing at me with unsure eyes.

That night, I thought back to how my parents disciplined me if I did something they didn't like. There were many times I was whipped with belts, extension cords, and switches from a nearby tree, all of which left large whelps and bruises on my skin. Once, I was even slapped so hard that blood gushed from my nose and ran down my face. My parents used their disciplinary techniques and the scars they left behind as a reminder of anything unacceptable to them. Overall, I learned my lessons, and that's all I want is for my sons to know right from wrong.

The next day, I received a call from the school. Our oldest son's friend noticed a bruise on his arm and asked what happened. Our son told him how he got in trouble for playing with matches. His friend was alarmed and thought it was important to report it to his counselor. She immediately contacted Social Services.

That evening, a family counselor knocked on our door, her expression a mix of sternness and concern. "Mr. Anderson," she said, calm but firmly, "I was informed about an incident that took place in your home yesterday. Can you tell me what happened?"

"My boys were playing with some matches and set some papers on fire. They didn't know how dangerously close they came to hurting themselves or burning down our house. I had to teach them a lesson so they wouldn't ever do that again."

The counselor stared at me in disbelief and shook her head, her disapproval evident on her face. "Your disciplinary methods are not acceptable, sir," she said.

"This matter has been reported to your command. You will be required to attend counseling."

After she left, I had to sit down and process what had happened. I was only doing what I had been taught, using the same disciplinary actions that my parents used on me, and I turned out fine. I'm a good dad and husband. *What did I do wrong?* I thought.

The military did not take this situation lightly. I was told to report to my commanding officer. Stern-faced and unyielding, he mandated that Annette and I attend family counseling. The sessions peeled back the layers of my upbringing, revealing the brutal legacy of discipline passed down through generations.

"Abe, you need to change," Annette said softly one night, her hand resting on mine, "for the sake of our children."

"You're right, Annette." The weight of my actions seemed to be pressing down on me.

Annette explained that her upbringing was a world apart from mine. Her parents, although strict, chose to spank her gently on the hands or buttocks or to scold her firmly. Afterward, they calmly explained why she was disciplined and ended their conversation with a hug and reassurances of their love. Annette firmly emphasized this was the technique she wanted to use on our children.

"Annette, this is a sharp contrast from what I am used to. But since your approach of using hugs and words of love seemed to foster respect and understanding from our children, I'm willing to try."

Annette smiled and embraced me.

That night, we turned to the Bible, seeking guidance and understanding. Slowly, I began to learn new ways to correct our children, ways that didn't leave them scarred and terrified. It was a long journey, filled with moments of doubt and struggle, but gradually, we found a path forward that we both agreed on. A path of love, understanding, and compassion.

Later, I discovered that my parents' disciplinary methods mirrored those they had endured in their childhoods. I also realized a chilling parallel in the harsh control tactics of slave masters, a legacy of pain passed down through generations. Without questioning, I had adopted the same severe approach with our children.

I'm so grateful that Annette spoke up and told me what I was doing was wrong. I needed to break these negative habits that were harmful to my children and family. My wife was patient with me and was willing to help guide me in disciplining our children with love based on God's word. In the process, we began to heal the wounds of the past, building a future for our children free from the shadows of fear and pain.

SEEKING COMFORT IN A BOTTLE

Military life was sometimes tough on us as a young family, especially when I was still learning how to be a husband and family man. I began to find that the stress of the job began to get to me. Before long, I was hanging out with the boys at the club every weekend, drinking more and more and coming home late. This is not where I thought my life would be. I had high hopes for myself, but my poor choices were negatively impacting my ability to function effectively in my home.

These behaviors were common for some military guys to help pass the time. However, this was not acceptable. I loved my wife and children more than anything in the world, and I did not want to disappointment them. In order to save my marriage, I had to stop drinking and get back on track.

My wife had expressed to me numerous times that she was not happy with these new habits I had picked up. I could see the hurt and pain in her eyes every time she spoke to me about my drinking, but I brushed it off initially and defended myself.

"I'm really not drinking that much, Annette. I've got this under control."

But seeing the disappointment on her face day after day was killing me. But I wasn't sure how to fix the situation.

One day, Annette said, "We need to talk."

These were the four words I used to dread hearing. However, I knew I needed to sit down and listen to her. I had to open my heart and mind to whatever she expressed to me without being defensive.

During our conversation, Annette expressed her concern that I was becoming a borderline alcoholic, drinking every weekend with my friends. She told me she felt I was not putting our family's needs first. She was right! And as a husband and father, my behaviors and choices were unacceptable. I knew I needed to get my life straight and show my wife and family through my actions that they were the most important people in my life. They needed to come first, not my personal desires.

"Annette, I'm so sorry that I've disappointed you with my drinking. I thought I had a handle on this, but apparently I don't. I admit that I've been drinking excessively, and I can see that it hurts you, and that's the last thing that I ever wanted to happen. I think I just let the influence of others and the stress of my job get the best of me. I love you and our kids and want to do right by you."

She looked at me for a long time, then told me everything would be alright. "Abe, I love you, and I can assure you that I'm going to do everything I can to help you fight this battle against alcoholism. You're not in this alone. There will be some tough times ahead, but we serve a mighty God who will help us get through this. We're not waiting. We're going to start today, right now!"

My wife picked up her anointing oil, rubbed it on my forehead, and prayed a powerful prayer. With lifted hands, she cried out to the Lord, asking God to deliver me from the bondage of alcoholism. She cried out, declaring that I would be saved before leaving England.

While she prayed, I closed my eyes, focusing on her prayers, accepting the challenge to be the man she had married, the man who loved her and wanted to protect her and our children. I was willing to do anything to save our marriage. It was a very moving moment. I felt something stir deep in my soul and had no doubt God would help me surrender to him so I could abstain from drinking alcohol. Afterward, we embraced and talked for quite some time.

Later that night, as I lay in bed, I prayed about my life, "Lord, I've been making a lot of mistakes lately, doing things that have been hurtful to my wife and our family, and exhibiting behaviors that are unbecoming of a man of God. I'm determined to make things better for all of us, and I really want to change my ways. Please help me to recommit my life to you, Lord. Help me change my behaviors so they are pleasing and acceptable to you and my wife. Thank you, Lord. Amen!"

A LIFE-CHANGING MOMENT

Over time, I began making some serious changes in my life and worked hard to turn things around. Annette and my family meant more to me than anything in this world. So, I stopped hanging out with my friends and quit going to the club to drink.

I couldn't stop thinking about the night Annette rubbed anointing oil on my forehead and prayed for me, declaring that I would be saved before we left England. Since I was scheduled to change duty stations soon, I needed to accept Christ in my life—not just because Annette asked me to, but because I wanted to be saved. I wanted to give my life to Christ. I needed Him in my life. I was not complete without the Lord. Having Him in my life would help me to be a better man and make better decisions. I was determined to be the husband and father that God created me to be. *How could I not surrender to Him when He saved my life and marriage?* I thought.

Later that night while I was taking a bath, my wife walked in with a serious look on her face and said, "Abraham, if you want to give your life to Christ Jesus, recite these words: 'Dear Lord Jesus, I am a sinner, and I ask for your forgiveness. I believe you died for my sins and rose from the dead. I turn from my sins and invite you to come into my heart and life. I want to trust and follow you as my Lord and Savior. Amen.'"

In that very private, intense moment, I repeated the prayer and felt an incredible transformation. I became a new creation in Christ Jesus, marking a profound new beginning in my life. I began to cultivate a personal relationship with God, starting each morning by thanking Him for His mercy and grace and for granting me another day of life.

After this spiritual experience, 1 John 2:5 (NIV) resonated deeply with me: "But if anyone obeys His word, love for God is truly made complete in them." Amen! This scripture encapsulated the essence of my newfound faith and commitment to living a life in obedience to His word.

MILITARY LIFE: FROM ONE DUTY STATION TO ANOTHER

A few years later, I was reassigned to Mechanicsburg, PA for two years. We were excited that we would be returning to the United States and be near our family, who were only an hour or so away. We found it very uplifting to spend more time with our families. Our children had the opportunity to interact with their cousins and grandparents. This reunion of our families was very much needed and was refreshing for our marriage since we had time to visit with our parents and siblings. We were able to attend the churches we had grown up in and spend more time with our families.

Sunsets and New Beginnings—Hawaii Bound

After being transferred from one duty station to another, I was thrilled when I learned my next duty station would be in Honolulu, Hawaii. This is the duty station every soldier dreams of being assigned to, with its grand palm trees, beautiful sandy beaches, crystal blue water, warm weather, fresh seafood, and a multicultural mix of beautiful, friendly people from all over the world.

My wife and I transitioned easily to living in Hawaii. We liked our new military home with three bedrooms and all its amenities. The kids attended a nearby elementary school and learned about the Hawaiian culture. It was nice meeting other military couples. We would often hang out with them. We thought it was important to stay connected with people of faith. So, after a while, we joined the Word of Life Christian Center Hawaii. My wife even sang in the choir and was a part of the Praise and Worship team. We enjoyed fellowshipping with other military families.

I was stationed at Tripler Army Medical Center, a beautiful and majestic facility with a bright coral façade that was built on top of a hill overlooking Honolulu. It stood out from all the other buildings on the island.

My duties at Tripler as a noncommissioned officer were to support the soldiers under me to ensure they met all of their physical fitness tests, Military Occupational Specialty (MOS) training which helps them to become experts in their chosen field, and any other important activities they were required to do. I also worked at Fort Shafter, a few miles from Tripler.

FROM ALOHA TO AGONY

Our happy life in Hawaii took a troubling turn when I started to experience severe and sometimes uncontrollable hiccups that affected my concentration to think or reason, and it caused confusion to where I lacked the desire to even work out. Each time they would flare up, I would go to the doctor. I couldn't understand what was happening to my body. After having these symptoms for approximately a year, I was diagnosed with gastroesophageal reflux disease, commonly known as GERD. They explained this occurs when stomach acid flows into the tube that connects my mouth and stomach. I was given antacids to control the symptoms.

When I told my wife what the doctor said, she commented that, based on her experience as a registered nurse, she wasn't sure if this was an accurate diagnosis.

I thought this beautiful, tropical island would bring us nothing but pure happiness. However, my hiccups persisted and worsened. My wife grew increasingly concerned and suggested I see a neurologist. So, I scheduled an appointment with one.

When we arrived at the neurologist's office, it seemed cold and sterile, amplifying my unease. The doctor walked in a few minutes later, and his gaze met mine. He had a hint of concern yet seemed clinically detached when he said, "Abraham, I'm worried about your persistent symptoms and the period of time you've been experiencing this anomaly." Glancing down at his chart, then locking eyes with me, he uttered "We need to have an MRI done today."

The MRI

The doctor seemed so concerned that I thought it was best for me to know for sure what was going on with my body. So, I went into the waiting room, changed into the hospital gown, and was then escorted into the exam room. As I lay down on the table, my heart and mind were racing. I couldn't believe how nervous I was. But I knew the results could impact my whole life.

The radiologist tech injected something clear into my veins. She explained it was a contrast liquid that would help to improve the quality of the images of my brain more clearly and help the doctor determine what was going on.

My mind wandered as I glanced around the cold room. "Lord, I pray nothing negative is revealed in the scans she captures, but if it is, Lord, I pray you will be with me all the way and that you will heal me."

The technologist began to rattle off instructions. "Mr. Anderson, once we start, please lie very still. Try to relax while you're inside the machine. If you move, it may distort the images, and we will have to do all of this again. If you experience any difficulty during the screening, let me know by pressing this button," she said, handing me the button attached to a long tube. "Don't worry; although you can't see me, I will be monitoring you during the scan and communicating with you via the speakers inside the MRI machine. Do you have any questions?"

I shook my head.

"Okay, let's get started," she said, and the table began to slowly slide into the huge, cylindrical chamber. I lay as still as I could, taking long, deep breaths. Soon, the machine's relentless loud, clanging, and knocking sounds increased my rising anxiety.

"Hold your breath, and don't move!"

I inhaled deeply, then held my breath, determined not to have to repeat these scans. The constant pinging and hammering of the machine, combined with my anxiety, made it difficult to lie still and hold my breath as instructed. This whole experience was nerve-wracking. At times, it felt like my lungs were going to burst from the lack of oxygen. My heart seemed to be pounding louder than the noise created by the MRI machine.

"Okay! You can breathe now!"

Finally allowed to breathe, I gasped for air, filling my lungs as much as I could.

Then, she quickly said again, "Hold your breath, don't move!" These directions were repeated numerous times.

What are they seeing? I wondered. I pray there are no abnormalities. I'm not sure how much time has passed by, I thought, *but it seems like this MRI is taking forever. I'm sure it's been at least thirty minutes I've been lying in here. Why is this taking so long? Have they spotted something?*

After an hour or so, the pinging and banging noises finally stopped, and the technologist's voice echoed in the chamber, saying, "You can breathe now! We are done. You did great, Mr. Anderson. Thank you!" And the table slowly slid out, away from the tight chamber walls.

CLINGING TO HOPE: AWAITING THE RESULTS

It seemed like an eternity as we waited for the results, even though it was only an hour later before the neurologist told us the results of my MRI. I was told to come in the following day for a pre-op to complete bloodwork and have another scan done.

Afterward, the doctor told me he saw an abnormality but wanted to wait to speak with me and my wife about the MRI results.

The nurse from the neurologist's office called my wife right away, requesting we both be present when the doctor reviews the MRI results. I tried to stay calm as we waited, but it was emotionally challenging for me.

As we sat in his office, I was filled with so much anxiety that dread began overtaking me as if it were a snake coiling in the pit of my stomach. My heart was beating ferociously against my chest as I tried desperately to calm down.

We were completely unprepared for the bombshell—***massive brain tumor***. Even if I considered emergency surgery, I struggled to fathom the gravity of the potential risks the doctor outlined. A stroke, speech or memory issues, loss of leg strength, paralysis, brain swelling, or a blood clot—these were just some of the possibilities. The most chilling part was when he said I could even lose my life during the procedure. Despite emphasizing a 92 percent survival rate, I couldn't shake the overwhelming uncertainty. Is it worth the risk? *I just don't know*, I thought, feeling overwhelmed.

Grappling with the Unthinkable

The long drive home was a silent descent into the unknown. My wife's worry was palpable, and I felt a desperate need to comfort her, to assure her that I was strong and would get through this— more importantly, that I was a man of faith. But even as I tried to speak, doubt gnawed at the edges of my resolve, so I sat quietly, trying desperately to find the words that would calm my bride, but they eluded me.

Finally, Annette broke the silence. "Look, I'm just as shocked and concerned as you are, but we can't let fear control us. Fear and faith cannot coexist. The Lord reminds us in Isaiah 41:10 NIV, "So, do not fear, for I am with you." We have to cling to God's words and not give in to fear. We must believe God in 2 Timothy 1:7, New King James Version when He says, "For God has not given us a spirit of fear, but of power and of love and of a sound mind." So, we have to trust that He will see you through this, Abe. We will do whatever it takes to save your life, but above all, we will rely on God's word. I love you, and I need you here with me. Our family needs you! We won't even entertain the possibility of death—not at all! Do you hear me, Abe?" she said firmly, looking at me with a steadfast, unwavering gaze.

"Yes," I said nodding. Her words rang true as if throwing me a lifeline in this storm of uncertainty. "I will be fine," I whispered aloud, attempting to reassure myself, as well as my wife.

"You've got to trust Him, Abe. He will bring you through this, but you must believe that He can."

I smiled and looked longingly at my wife! I knew she was right and that she would fight for me through her powerful prayers to the sovereign God we served. She is my angel warrior, a God-fearing woman who takes everything to God in prayer.

I prayed silently to God. "I am a covenant man of God who loves you, Lord, who worships and adores you. I faithfully pay my tithes and serve within the church. So, why is this happening to me?" I didn't want doubt to cloud my mind and get in the way of me keeping my focus on God, my redeemer. I shook my head back and forth in an attempt to dislodge negative thoughts. "Lord, please capture these negative thoughts and remove them from my mind. Help me to stay focused on You. Please be with me and my wife as we navigate these difficult times ahead. I trust you, Lord."

PREPARING FOR WARFARE

Annette and I believe in the power of prayer and God's promises. As we prepared for my pending surgery, we gathered scriptures for healing and verses to remind us of God's promises. We read our Bible verses together, prayed, and listened to worship songs to keep us uplifted.

We could not go into this battle alone; we needed the support of our faith community. So, we contacted Pastor Art and Kuna Sepulveda from Word of Life Church in Hawaii and other pastors, elders, and members of our church who believed that God could heal me. We reached out to family and friends and asked them to pray for my healing. It took some effort to mobilize such a massive prayer group, but everyone agreed to pray for me, Annette, and our family.

Now that we had surrounded ourselves with prayer warriors, we prayed several Bible verses as we prepared for my pending surgery and hospital stay. These powerful verses from the New King James Version of the Bible kept me encouraged:

- "I shall not die, but live, and declare the works of the Lord," (Psalm 118:17).

- "If you diligently heed the voice of the Lord your God and do what is right in His sight, give ear to His commandments and keep all his statutes, I will put none of the diseases on you which I have brought on the Egyptians. For I am the LORD who heals you," (Exodus 15:26).

- "Let us therefore come boldly to the throne of grace, that we may obtain mercy and find grace to help in time of need," (Hebrew 4:16).

- "The effective, fervent prayer of a righteous man avails much," (James 5:16).

- "Therefore I say to you, whatever things you ask when you pray, believe that you receive them, and you will have them," (Mark 11:24).

- "For I will restore health to you and heal you of your wounds,' says the Lord,'" (Jeremiah 30:17).

When you're reading these verses when you're sick and in need of God's mercy and grace, they seem to carry a special meaning and have a sense of urgency.

The Love of Family & Friends

We weren't sure how long I would be in the hospital, and Annette wanted to be by my side every step of the way. So, she contacted her mother, who was stateside, to see if she would come to Hawaii and help with our three, elementary-age children. Her mother didn't hesitate. She assured Annette that she would be there, and within a few days, she flew to Hawaii and was ready to assist as promised.

Knowing that our family and friends were coming to our aid really meant the world to us. Now that our army of prayer warriors was assembled, we were ready to deal with whatever was coming next—a war against the unknown.

THE BATTLE BEGINS

Surgery #1

I checked into the hospital, ready to undergo brain surgery. My wife and I talked and prayed as we waited in my room. Soon, the surgeon came in and greeted us.

"Mr. and Mrs. Anderson," he said, looking at us intently. "There are a few things I need to go over with you about the surgery."

My heart began pounding harder as I waited for him to discuss the procedure. Although I thought I was mentally and emotionally prepared for this day, it was still unnerving knowing they would be operating on my brain. I took a few deep breaths, trying to calm my nerves.

"The surgery will be lengthy because of the tedious task of removing the tumor from the base of your brain," he explained. "We expect the surgery to last approximately eighteen hours."

My wife and I glanced at each other when we heard "eighteen hours." *Wow!* I thought. *This is really going to be much more involved than I could ever imagine if it's going to take eighteen hours to remove this tumor.*

Looking at my wife, he continued, "So, I don't want you to be too concerned if Abraham is in surgery longer than that. This procedure takes time. I'll have someone update you from time to time, Mrs. Anderson. Any questions?"

"No!" we both said in unison.

"Just please take care of my husband," Annette said, "and bring him back to me."

"That's our intention. We'll do our best," he said as he exited the room.

I was wheeled into the operating room. The surgeon explained what would occur during surgery; his words were a blur in my mind. I was told to count backward from 100 and was soon fast asleep. Unbeknownst to me, while I was still sedated, the hours ticked by—five hours, ten hours, fifteen hours, then *eighteen hours had passed*.

Finally, the doctor came out to update my wife on how the surgery was going. "We had planned to remove all of the tumor from Abraham's brain; unfortunately, even after eighteen hours, we were not able to. At this point, we will continue monitoring him in the hospital for a few days up to a week or so. If he remains stable, he can go home and rest. But then, he'll need to come back in a month so we can remove the rest of the tumor.

Nevertheless, that plan quickly unraveled. Just eight hours post-surgery, my wife noticed the area on the back of my neck was swelling. It was the size of an orange, and blood was seeping through the sutures. Annette grabbed the call button, pressing it repeatedly as she waited for the nurse to come in.

When the nurse dashed through the door of my room, Annette said, "Get the surgeon right now! Something's wrong! The pig skin covering my husband's brain is filling with blood, and there's a pool of blood on his pillow."

The doctor came rushing into my hospital room and began examining me. He discovered that my brain was hemorrhaging. Without hesitation, everyone sprang into action, wheeling me quickly back to the operating room for emergency surgery.

Annette immediately switched into prayer-warrior mode, interceding on my behalf and praying to God to send angels to surround and protect me. Despite the grim circumstances, she stood firm on God's Words, believing His promises to heal me. She reached out to our pastors, congregation, family, and friends, rallying them to pray for a miracle on my behalf. Annette contacted other churches and prayer centers to pray for me.

Surgery #2- Emergency Surgery

For **_ten long hours_**, the surgeon worked feverishly to stop the hemorrhaging on my neck. The surgery appeared to be successful. After being monitored in the recovery room for a while, I was wheeled back to my room. My wife was relieved to see me. I don't remember much about it because I was still groggy.

Surgery #3- Second Emergency Surgery

We thought I was out of the woods and that the emergency surgery had resolved the problem. However, a few days later, I had to undergo another emergency surgery because the bleeding in my brain persisted.

During this surgery, my heart stopped. No heartbeat! Nothing! I had coded! But behind the scenes, God was working His miracles, showing the doctors and the medical team that He was in charge.

Later, the doctor told us about how my heart stopped during my surgery but miraculously started beating again on its own. As a precaution, he placed me on life support. This surgery lasted for ***eight hours*** and was indeed a test of faith and endurance.

The Final Surgery #4

I was prepped and ready for what was supposed to be the final surgery to remove the remaining portion of the tumor. After ***twelve hours*** slowly ticked by as I lay on the operating room bed, the surgeon informed the medical team they needed to stop working on me because they didn't want to risk my life.

When I woke up groggy and disoriented, Annette was there by my side holding my hand and smiling. She looked so angelic, my prayer warrior.

"The surgeon's coming to talk to us," she said, her voice steady, yet I glimpsed the worry in her eyes.

The doctor walked in. "I'm sorry, Mr. and Mrs. Anderson, but we couldn't remove the entire tumor," he began with a disheartened tone. "Your blood pressure kept spiking dangerously high during the procedure. We had to leave a small portion behind to avoid any further complications, such as a stroke."

I could see the disappointment in Annette's eyes, but she quickly masked it with determination. "What's next?" she asked.

"Given the circumstances, I recommend radiation therapy to target any remaining cancerous cells that may be lingering," he stated. "But, before you can start radiation, we'll need to fit you with a radiotherapy mesh mask to ensure precision during the treatment. It's designed to hold your head still during radiotherapy."

I nodded, trying to absorb all of this information. I felt like my brain was on overload. But I wanted to do everything I could to live and become whole again. Annette and I discussed the options the doctor shared with us. We prayed and put everything in God's hands.

RADIATION TREATMENT

The following week, I lay on a table in the Radiation Therapy room, somewhat intimidated by the large machine looming over my head. The radiotherapy technicians worked diligently as they molded the mesh mask to my face; its tight grip made me feel claustrophobic.

Soon, my radiation therapy began. It was a grueling ordeal. Every day for six weeks, Monday through Friday, I underwent thirty minutes of radiation treatments. I was exhausted! My body was weak, but my spirit clung to hope.

Extended Hospital Stay

Throughout my stay in the hospital, Annette was my unwavering rock. She screened every visitor who wanted to visit me. Her motto was clear, "No spectators allowed!" She didn't want anyone visiting me whose faith didn't speak life and healing. People who were not faith-driven and did not believe in God's saving grace or were not hopeful on my behalf were not permitted to see me.

"Not even my Colonel and Sergeant Major?" I asked, surprised.

"Not even them," Annette confirmed firmly. "They don't believe you can be healed, and I won't have that negativity around you."

My wife's fierce protection and unwavering faith were my anchors through this storm. I loved the way she guarded my physical and spiritual well-being.

After more than a month in the hospital, the toll on my body was immense. The multiple surgeries and extensive radiation treatments left me weak and bedridden. The physical strain was so overwhelming, and the emotional and mental exhaustion weighed heaviest on my mind. There were times I wasn't sure if I was going to survive, but I struggled to cling to God's promises.

However, Annette never wavered. "You're going to get through this," she would say, her eyes fierce with conviction.

My wife's belief in my recovery helped keep me going, even during the darkest days. The prolonged hospital stay was a trial of endurance, but with Annette by my side, it made it easier to hold onto hope. Her strength and faith became my lifeline, guiding me through the most trying time of my life.

THE FAITH TO FIGHT

Although I have no memory of this, when I was better, I was told that because of my extensive hospital stay and the limited progress I was making, I was placed on a ventilator and put in a medically induced coma. It seemed that my doctor didn't think I was going to make it, so he suggested that a priest come to pray for me and administer my last rites. My wife believed in the power of God and didn't want him to do that. However, the priest did give me the last rites when Annette was out of my hospital room.

When I came out of the coma, I was extremely weak and thought I was going to die. I remember thinking, *This can't be it. I'm not ready to leave Annette and our family.* A wave of helplessness washed over me, and depression and anxiety began to creep in.

Despite my physically weakened state, I wasn't ready to give up. I knew I had to fight back spiritually. With tears streaming down my face, I prayed fervently, asking God to strengthen me from head to toe. I took a deep breath, exhaled, and began speaking life over my body, repeatedly reciting Psalm 118:17 in the NKJV: "I shall not die, but live." Then, I prayed, "Lord, please strengthen and heal my body. Make me whole again." Weeks later, I was still clinging to life. My strength was slowly returning. "Thank you, Lord," I whispered. "I'm so glad I serve a God who listens to his sheep and answers their prayers."

Aloha to Hope: Witnessing God's Miracle Healing

After weeks in the hospital, the doctor came in to talk to me. "Mr. Anderson, we need to schedule you for another MRI so I can see if the radiation treatments were effective in shrinking your tumor."

"Okay," I said. The possibility of going home almost seemed foreign to me. Yet, I was excited. I had been in the hospital for so long and hadn't entered the doors of my own home, my sanctuary, in some time. I wasn't sure what it would feel like walking through those doors, laying in my own bed, eating my food, and sitting around talking with my wife, our kids, and family and friends.

Following the scan, the doctor went to talk to Annette. "Mrs. Anderson, will you come with me?"

"Why? What happened? What's wrong with Abe?" Annette said, anxious to find out what the doctor discovered.

"Look, I can't explain to you what the results reveal. I think it'll be best if you come look at it yourself." He gave no further hints as he walked briskly but quietly to the office; his expression was unreadable.

Anxiety was clearly etched on Annette's face as she followed, keeping up with his pace.

The doctor walked to the wall where the images of the scans were posted. He pointed to the initial MRI that revealed the massive brain tumor. Then, he pointed to the other screening that was just completed.

Bewildered, the doctor looked at my wife and said, "We never mix theology and science, but I have to admit there was a supreme being over this case. I've never seen anything like this. We know for a fact that we left a portion of the tumor there," he said, pointing at the scan. "But look, it's completely gone! There is no sign of residual tissue from the tumor in his head. There's no sign of it at all," he said, dismayed.

Annette's eyes filled with tears of joy and relief. She exhaled a long sigh of relief and quickly declared, "It was nothing but God! I told all of you from the beginning that God was going to remove my husband's tumor," she said, her faith vindicated in the face of medical impossibility. Then, she looked up to Heaven and whispered, "God, You *are* real! Thank you for your grace and mercy!" A beautiful smile quickly beamed across her face.

THROUGH SICKNESS AND HEALTH

When you're entirely dependent on your spouse, it deepens your appreciation for having someone who can stand in the gap for you. My wife, Annette, demonstrated her profound love by putting everything on hold to care for me from dawn until dusk.

During my darkest days and most challenging times, when I couldn't do anything for myself, Annette was there to feed me breakfast, lunch, and dinner. She assisted me to the bathroom daily and bathed me when the hospital nurses were too busy or overwhelmed. Annette walked with me up and down the halls to help strengthen my legs. She pushed my wheelchair to ensure I made it to my physical therapy sessions. At bedtime, she would get into bed with me and hold me until visiting hours were over.

Throughout my hospital stay, Annette was a constant presence, making sure everything went smoothly. She brought the kids to see me, which was immensely therapeutic for my soul. She instructed the nurses on each shift to play praise and worship music to help keep my mind focused on healing. Through all her actions during this trying time, Annette showed just how much she loved and cherished me and was committed to our wedding vows—for better or worse, in sickness and in health, so help me God.

Thinking of how amazing my wife is brings tears to my eyes. I know that I am a blessed man. Proverbs 18:22 in the New King James Version confirms it: "He who finds a wife finds a good thing, and obtains favor from the Lord." A man cannot attain anything better than a good wife. With confidence, I can boldly say that my wife is a woman of valor, strong and committed, capable of achieving anything she sets her mind to. She prayed me through the worst time of my life.

From Hospital to Home: Embracing a New Chapter

I was relieved when the doctor released me from the hospital and finally allowed me to go home. When I was admitted to the hospital, I had no idea I would have to endure four brain surgeries and stay there for over a month. With everything I'd been through and almost losing my life, I wasn't sure if I would ever return to the place I call my sanctuary—my home.

As I stepped through the doorway, I immediately felt the comfort it brought me. But then, anxiety began to overtake me. My heart pounded fiercely against my chest as a whirlwind of questions filled my mind. "Is my mind and body strong enough to do the things I need to do? Am I too weak to care for and protect my wife and family? Is my manhood going to be questioned? Can I fulfill my fatherly duties?"

As I walked further into my home, unhealthy thoughts continued to run rampant through my head. I quickly remembered a verse in the Bible that would help me calm my spirit: Philippians 4:6–7, "Be anxious for nothing, but in everything by prayer and supplication, with thanksgiving, let your requests be made known to God; and the peace of God, which surpasses all understanding, will guard your hearts and minds through Christ Jesus." After reciting this verse in my mind, I could feel my body relax a little. Then, I recited Philippians 4:13, reminding myself, "I can do all things through Christ who strengthens me." This helped me believe that I am capable of managing my daily responsibilities.

Faith and Family Sustained Me: My Mother-in-Law

My mother-in-law, Dorothy W. Spriggs, from Baltimore, Maryland, dropped everything to ensure our children were taken care of by assisting my wife during my hospitalization. She stepped in seamlessly, feeding the kids breakfast and dinner while the school took care of lunch. She prepared them for school, drove them to appointments and sports activities, and was gracious enough to entertain them until bedtime. Dorothy helped me stay on track by reminding me that God was not done with me yet and that I had kids to raise and a wife to support. Her sacrifice and unwavering faith were a beacon of hope during that difficult time. We were grateful that her husband, Reverend Franklin Spriggs, allowed her to stay and assist us for two months.

My Brother's Keeper

When my brother, Sylvester Anderson, heard about my surgery, he took a sabbatical from work and took time away from his family obligations to travel over four thousand miles to be by my side. The day he arrived, he walked into my hospital room, his face etched with concern and determination. Seeing him there, I felt a surge of strength and comfort. His presence made me feel special and supported. I truly believe that witnessing my healing process firsthand deepened his relationship with God.

My Siblings Rallied Support

My sisters and brothers—Marbin, Benjamin, Patricia, Joseph, Elise, Tinnie, and Joel—rallied in prayer as soon as they heard about my condition. We grew up believing in God's miraculous healing power, so they immediately contacted their church members, friends, other believers, and local prayer lines, asking them to pray for a miracle on my behalf.

THE STRENGTH OF THE CHURCH

After my recovery and release from the hospital, Pastor Art and Kuna Sepulveda, who had witnessed my miracle healing, requested that my wife and I share our testimony via video. He said that our story needed to be told because people needed to hear about the miracle that God performed in my life. I felt a wave of gratitude for the love, prayers, fasting, and anointing they had showered upon us.

They treated my family and me with the love of Christ with an outpouring of prayers, fasting, and anointing. This made me realize that they were the true shepherds of God's pasture, and they taught us how to be committed and steadfast in God's Word and to believe and stand on His Word. I grew stronger in the Word of God because of their leadership.

My wife and I were also supported by our church family and friends on the mainland. Along with their congregations, they were there for us through our season of darkness. I can truly say they stood in the gap for me and my family when we had doubts or uncertainties about the next phase in life.

God places people around you in your time of need, and He did that for us. We are forever grateful to our family and friends who dedicated their time and effort to help me heal and take care of our family.

Even though we struggled at times and wanted to give up, our faith remained strong and confident in the God we served. I am forever grateful to my children and wife for their steadfast love and support throughout my extensive illness and recovery.

There was no magic pill or secret potion that was responsible for restoring my health. It was solely by the grace and mercy of God that I was healed. I am living proof that God still performs miracles. The power of the Word of God, the Bible, brimming with hope, faith, and God's promises, kept me encouraged, along with the prayers of many family and friends. God is the only reason I had a successful recovery and was delivered from the brink of death. I am grateful to be alive today. All the glory belongs to Him!

A SECOND CHANCE

Months later, after my health crisis and rehabilitation, I returned to my military unit and, by the grace of God, completed all my duties without assistance. Passing my physical fitness tests with flying colors, I met every Army requirement.

A Legacy of Service in the United States Army

As I reflected on my military career, for someone who is athletically inclined and loves to work out daily, earning the Expert Field Medical Badge was a significant achievement. The Expert Field Medical Badge is the highest test of professional competence and physical endurance for a soldier medic in the United States Army. The test includes 144 hours of continuous operational events that challenge the mental and physical stamina, as well as the tactical and technical skills of a medical soldier.

Air Assault School, a 10-day course that teaches Air Assault techniques, is one of the most physically demanding courses I took in the Army, requiring extensive training and perseverance. I served as a First Sergeant with twenty-three years of active service, holding a leadership position as a senior noncommissioned officer in the United States Army.

Throughout my military career, I attended several managerial, supervisory, and leadership schools, which enhanced my ability to lead over five hundred soldiers. My technical skills and extensive experience at various military installations across the United States and Europe allowed me to interact with people from diverse backgrounds. My attributes clearly indicate that I am a goal-oriented, dedicated professional and a highly motivated self-starter and decision-maker. These experiences not only honed my leadership abilities but also enriched my understanding of cultural dynamics and teamwork.

Additionally, my technical skills encompass the following:

- **Operational Planning and Execution:** Proficient in developing and implementing strategic operational plans that ensure mission success and soldier readiness.

- **Training and Development:** Skilled in designing and conducting comprehensive training programs that enhance the tactical and technical proficiency of soldiers.

- **Crisis Management:** Experienced in managing high-pressure situations, making quick decisions, and maintaining composure during crises.

- **Communication:** Adept at clear and effective communication, both written and verbal, ensuring seamless coordination and information dissemination within the unit.

- **Mentorship:** Committed to mentoring junior soldiers, fostering their professional growth, and preparing them for future leadership roles.

- **Adaptability:** Adapted to various environments and challenges, consistently achieving objectives regardless of circumstances.

These attributes highlight my dedication to excellence, my motivation as a self-starter, and my decisive leadership style. For most of my military career, I scored 100 percent on my Army physical fitness test which earned me the physical fitness patch. In addition, I consistently ensured that over ninety-five soldiers were qualified in common tasks such as Military Occupational Specialty training, the Army physical fitness test, and soldier readiness.

Balancing Duty and Academic Success in the Military

While in the military, I wanted to pursue an undergraduate degree, but at the same time, I doubted whether or not I could afford it and whether I was smart enough. While trying to figure out what I was going to do and after talking to a few people, I discovered that the military would pay for my tuition. What more could I ask for? After weighing the pros and cons, I made the monumental decision to attend college. With newfound determination, I mustered up the courage to apply for my first college classes. I was excited and proud that I had made this important decision for my life. However, shortly after signing the required documents, anxiety, stress, and doubt began to cloud my mind. I questioned my decision to start college as past learning deficiencies resurfaced, haunting my thoughts.

In this moment of uncertainty, I turned to God's word for guidance and strength. I read and prayed on James 1:6–7 NIV states, "But when you ask, you must believe and not doubt, because the one who doubts is like a wave of the sea, blown and tossed by the wind. That person should not expect to receive anything from the Lord." Embracing this scripture, I declared and decreed over my situation, applying God's message to my life and believing that I could pass my classes and obtain a degree.

With faith and perseverance, I was able to complete my undergraduate and graduate degrees. In doing so, I set a positive example for my family and fellow soldiers, demonstrating the power of God's word, my faith and belief, and my resilience.

During my final duty station in the United States Army, I served as a Veterinary Food Inspector in the medical field in San Diego, CA. I had achieved the rank of First Sergeant and became eligible for promotion to

Sergeant Major. However, that meant transferring to the Sergeant Major Academy in Fort Bliss, Texas, for a year or more.

Because my wife had sacrificed so much for me during my years of service and my extensive illness, I felt obligated to put in for retirement from the United States Army. It was time for Annette to do what she had always dreamed of—completing her master's degree in nursing and obtaining a nurse practitioner degree.

Serving in the military is unlike any other job you can imagine. I will always be proud and grateful for the experiences and opportunities I was given in the United States Army while serving and protecting my country! I will cherish this incredible journey for the rest of my life.

After retiring from the military, I dedicated twelve years to educating young minds as a Junior Reserve Officer Training Corps instructor at Crawford High School in San Diego, California. There, I taught Military Science, Drill and Ceremony, Leadership Development, Physical Fitness as mandated by the United States Army and the San Diego Unified School District's curriculum requirements to shape future leaders with the same skills and dedication that had defined my career.

AN ENDURING LOVE AND ETERNAL COMMITMENT

My life would have been drastically different had I not met Annette, the lady and love of my life, over fifty years ago. Even though we struggled at times through life's hills and valleys and wanted to give up, we chose to stay together, committed to seeing what the future holds. The only way we accomplished this is because our faith remained strong and confident in the God we served.

Some marriages might have crumbled under the strain of what we endured, but ours emerged stronger. My near-death experience and long recovery was a life-changing event that actually fortified our marital bond. If it had not been for my God-fearing wife standing diligently on the Word, I might have faced a different outcome. Annette was my voice when I couldn't speak, my legs when I couldn't walk, and my mind when I couldn't express my thoughts. She was, and is, my everything!

Even as Annette and I grow old together, she will forever be the lady of my life. No matter what challenges come our way, we are determined to hold on to God's unchanging hand. We are determined to uphold our marriage vows and be obedient to the Bible. We proudly stand as a true representation of Genesis 2:24, "Therefore a man shall leave his father and his mother and hold fast to his wife, and they shall become one flesh," (English Standard Version).

As a result, being a man of God, I am committed to holding tight to the love of my life. I will love and cherish Annette Anderson for the rest of my life!

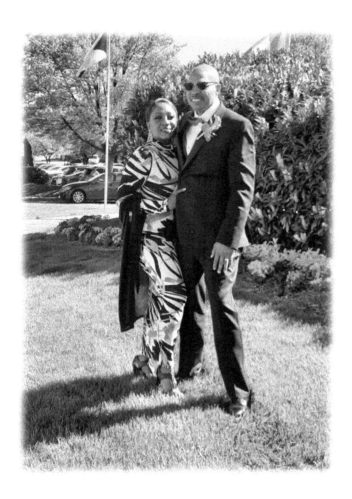

SUMMARY

In summary, I am living proof that if you put your faith in motion, God will perform miracles. My battle with a massive tumor on my brain and near-death experience is a testament to God's merciful healing. Hebrews 10:23 says, "Let us hold firmly to the confession of our hope without wavering, since He who promised is faithful," (Evangelical Heritage Version).

No matter the struggles or how difficult the situation may seem, don't lose hope! Whether you're facing health issues, dealing with the pain of loss, the weight of financial burdens, or the anguish of broken relationships, know that you are not alone. Battling depression or feeling overwhelmed by life's demands can make the journey seem insurmountable. Yet, through faith and perseverance, you can find the strength to overcome these obstacles and emerge stronger. Trust in God and His word, for He promises to guide you and provide the strength needed to endure and triumph over every hardship.

When you read the following Bible verses from the New King James Version, seek God's promises in His word. I pray they will provide you with comfort and guidance as you navigate life's challenges. Most of all, I implore you to trust and believe the Lord will be with you always.

1. **When You Are Ill:**

   - James 5:14–15: "Is anyone among you sick? Let him call for the elders of the church, and let them pray over him, anointing him with oil in the name of the Lord. And the prayer of faith will save the sick, and the Lord will raise him up."

2. **When You Need Guidance:**

   - Proverbs 3:5–6: "Trust in the LORD with all your heart, and lean not on your own understanding; in all your ways acknowledge Him, and He shall direct your paths."

3. **When You Are Sad:**

   - Psalm 34:18: "The LORD is near to those who have a broken heart, and saves such as have a contrite spirit."

4. **When You Are Lonely:**

   - Deuteronomy 31:6: "Be strong and of good courage, do not fear nor be afraid of them; for the

LORD your God, He is the One who goes with you. He will not leave you nor forsake you."

5. **When You Feel Weak:**

    - Isaiah 40:29: "He gives power to the weak, and to those who have no might He increases strength."

6. **When You Are Worried:**

    - Philippians 4:6–7: "Be anxious for nothing, but in everything by prayer and supplication, with thanksgiving, let your requests be made known to God; and the peace of God, which surpasses all understanding, will guard your hearts and minds through Christ Jesus."

7. **When You Are Afraid:**

    - Psalm 23:4: "Yea, though I walk through the valley of the shadow of death, I will fear no evil; for You are with me; Your rod and Your staff, they comfort me."

8. **When You Are Depressed:**

    - Psalm 42:11: "Why are you cast down, O my soul? And why are you disquieted within me? Hope in God; for I shall yet praise Him, the help of my countenance and my God."

9. **When You Are Struggling with Loss:**

   - Matthew 5:4: "Blessed are those who mourn, for they shall be comforted."

10. **When You Are Stressed:**

    - 1 Peter 5:7: "Casting all your care upon Him, for He cares for you."

11. **When Experiencing Marital Problems:**

    - Ephesians 4:2–3: "With all lowliness and gentleness, with longsuffering, bearing with one another in love, endeavoring to keep the unity of the Spirit in the bond of peace."

12. **When You Need Strength:**

    - Philippians 4:13: "I can do all things through Christ who strengthens me."

13. **When You Seek Peace:**

    - John 14:27: "Peace I leave with you, my peace I give to you; not as the world gives do I give to you. Let not your heart be troubled, neither let it be afraid."

14. **When You Need Comfort:**

    - 2 Corinthians 1:3–4: "Blessed be the God and Father of our Lord Jesus Christ, the Father of mercies and God of all comfort, who comforts us in all our tribulation."

15. **When You Need Hope:**

- Romans 15:13: "Now may the God of hope fill you with all joy and peace in believing, that you may abound in hope by the power of the Holy Spirit."

16. **When You Need Encouragement:**

- Isaiah 41:10: "Fear not, for I am with you; be not dismayed, for I am your God. I will strengthen you, yes, I will help you, I will uphold you with my righteous right hand."

17. **When You Are Confused:**

- James 1:5: "If any of you lacks wisdom, let him ask of God, who gives to all liberally and without reproach, and it will be given to him."

18. **When You Feel Overwhelmed:**

- Psalm 61:2: "From the end of the earth I will cry to You, when my heart is overwhelmed; lead me to the rock that is higher than I."

19. **When You Are Seeking Assurance:**

- Romans 8:28: "And we know that all things work together for good to those who love God, to those who are the called according to His purpose."

20. **When You Need Faith:**

- Hebrews 11:1: "Now faith is the substance of things hoped for, the evidence of things not seen."

RESOURCES

Alcoholics Anonymous
https://www.aa.org

Military.com
https://www.military.com › Spouse › Relationships

Military OneSource (.mil)
https://www.militaryonesource.mil › plan-to-move › pc...

Military Support for Families Assigned to New Bases

National Military Family Association
https://www.militaryfamily.org › Blog

Operation We Are Here
https://www.operationwearehere.com › military marriage

Substance Abuse and Mental Health Services (SAMHSA'S) National Helpline
www.samhsa.gov

ABOUT THE AUTHOR

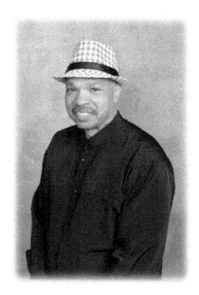

Abraham Anderson, number seven of nine siblings, was born and raised in Baltimore, Maryland. He attended Mergenthaler Senior vocational technical High School and majored in Business Administration. He has an Associate Degree in General Studies from Central Texas College, a Bachelor of Science in Psychology and a minor in Management from Columbia College, and a Master of Science in Administration from Central Michigan University.

Abraham served 23 years in the United States Army as a Veterinary Food Inspector, Medical field. His rank of retirement was First Sergeant.

After serving in the Military, he became a Junior Reserve Officer Training Corp instructor at Crawford High School -San Diego Unified School District, California, for twelve years. He taught Military Science, Drill and Ceremony, Leadership Development, curri-culum requirements, and Physical Fitness programs as mandated by the San Diego School District and United States Army.

Abraham married his high school sweetheart, Annette Anderson, and together they have three adult children Jamal, Brandon Anderson, and Tiyauna Zambrano. They have been married for forty years and currently reside in Southern California.

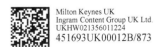
Milton Keynes UK
Ingram Content Group UK Ltd.
UKHW021356011224
451693UK00012B/873